Suicide Headaches, Short Trips and Saved Lives

By Stephen Young

ISBN: 978-1515216247

*For Kapil, Eberth, "Roger," "Jack,"
and all my fellow travelers*

Table of Contents

1. 4' 33"

The slight sensation of pressure concentrated at the center top of my left eye socket woke me up at about 3 a.m. It was early November of 2012. The feeling wasn't precisely pain, yet, but a quick succession of thoughts and emotions got me out of bed. First was panic at the thought of another series of headaches, followed by the memory that there was a way to deal with it now. Then slight amusement: it could well be a mildly psychedelic holiday season.

Dull, light discomfort throbbed above my eye as I tried to rise quietly without waking my wife. Compressed in a small spot about the size of a sunflower seed, the feeling of pressure was still causing a near-Proustian series of mental imagery and physical remembrances. The mystery of the headaches, the attempts to stay ahead of them with conventional medication that always failed, the feeling that someone had driven a sand-encrusted nail through my skull before proceeding to twist it slowly, the hours of simply pacing the floor while waiting for the pain to pass, and then the near-mystical quest that ended with a tool to address the condition.

I crept downstairs, entered the garage and found the stepladder that allowed me to access the highest shelf of the tool cabinet. I opened up the box that I hadn't looked at for about 3 years. The dried mushrooms were still there and they looked OK. I broke off a very small piece of one stem – maybe the size of a sunflower seed. I popped it under my tongue, still thinking about the past, but also fairly certain that the pressure would pass quickly. I would be back to sleep soon.

2. Metal Machine Music

When I awoke with the same sensation about ten years earlier, the initial panic didn't subside – it gave way to a more intense fear. I felt the kind of physical sinking deep in my stomach that seemed to parallel being startled by something grossly threatening in a personal space – like seeing a tarantula on your pillow when first waking.

I was afraid. I didn't want it to start again.

I had noticed the headaches when I was younger, starting in my early 20s, but into my late 20s the pain became increasingly intense and prolonged. It seemed like the episodes didn't just go away after a couple months, as they had in the past. In the year 1999, when I was 32 years old, the pain just dragged on throughout winter and into the spring.

A visit to my doctor that year revealed the diagnosis. I had told him I assumed a sinus infection woke me up just about every night at 3 a.m. with an intense pain above my eye. I told him I had been taking decongestants, but they took at least an hour to work, sometimes much longer.

The doctor asked a series of questions that seemed focused on the very narrow spot of discomfort. He asked if the eye with the pain turned bloodshot while the other stayed clear. He asked if one nostril dripped on the side of the headache as it subsided. I said yes and mentioned another peculiarity: at the same time my nostril starting dripping a few tears would be shed, but just from the eye that was aching, not from the other eye.

"Cluster headaches," he said, with perhaps a bit of pride at a difficult diagnosis. He noted that he was also one of the rare people who got them. The tears from a single eye and nasal drip from one nostril as relief returned are among the unique symptoms of cluster headaches, he said while tapping a spot on his own skull right above his eye.

9

The intense pain is caused by blood vessel dilation which creates pressure on the trigeminal nerve above the eye, but the actual cause of the dilation is unknown, though current research suggests the problem might be controlled by the Hypothalamus region of the brain. Sometimes the episodes of pain are referred to as "suicide headaches" due to their intolerable intensity. Relatively few people suffer from them (only about 1 in 10,000), and there didn't seem to be a whole lot known about them at the time, except that some foods and drugs tended to aggravate their intensity.

I thought it was odd that they were called cluster headaches, as they seemed pinpointed in such a precise part of the head. The doctor explained that the word "cluster" did not refer to locations of headaches, but instead to frequency of headaches. Sufferers tend to get them in cycles over several months, often for about three months at a time. The headaches are usually less intense and frequent at the beginning of the cycle, but frequency and intensity increase, usually peaking out at the middle of the cycle (or at about six weeks into a typical cycle).

That was essentially the pattern my headaches had followed. When I first noticed them, they would happen a couple times a week, and would be more of an irritation than a health crisis. But as the weeks went on, the headaches would appear four times a week, and then, finally, daily. In the height of the cluster, the pain was intense and long-lasting, sometimes persisting close to three hours at a time. The sensation – a grinding pressure in a small spot right above my left eye that seemed to increase in exponential waves of intensity even as I imagined they couldn't get worse – responded to no standard analgesic that I tried. But then the headaches would start fading to a few times a week, ending as they started, as a weekly irritation.

While they generally did not last beyond a few hours, my headaches almost always arrived at 3 a.m., leaving me sleep deprived, physically-drained and in a state something like a pain hangover that lasted through much of the following day.

I learned I am atypical among the atypical who get the headaches. Most poor souls with cluster headaches experience a cycle annually. Mine seemed to appear every three years or so, sometimes more frequently. I would go years without thinking about the headaches, almost allowing myself to forget, but they always came back. I can't imagine the dread of knowing it was coming each and every year, also knowing there was nothing I could do about them. Some people have the headaches consistently without interruption. Trying to envision that kind of experience makes the nickname "suicide headaches" not just comprehensible, but chillingly rational.

It was good to know what was happening, but there wasn't much to be done. The doctor gave me a list of foods to avoid – aged cheeses and pickled vegetables that were likely to have mold, and some food additives like MSG. He said if I consumed alcohol, caffeine or tobacco, I should quit while the headaches were active. Don't take conventional pain medications, he said, as they could aggravate the condition. And he gave me a prescription for Imitrex, a medication commonly used for migraine headaches (which cause completely different symptoms than cluster headaches).

The thought of a medication that addressed the pain was a relief, until I actually tried the medication. At first the Imitrex did seem to push back at the pain, but I soon had a case of the bedspins that rivaled memories from my most irresponsible alcohol use. At some point I wasn't sure if the pain had disappeared or merely been overshadowed by nausea. Worse, about eight hours later, the headache returned in a phenomenon known as "rebound." Cluster headaches are notorious for coming back quickly with a vengeance if merely suppressed.

I gave the Imitrex one more chance, but the bed spun again. By that time, the cycle was ending, so I just toughed out the last few weeks.

3. Golden Hours

I didn't think about them again until 2004, when the next headache cycle started. I had a different family doctor by then, who didn't know much about cluster headaches. She referred me to a neurologist, who wouldn't be able to see me for a month, roughly when the headaches would be approaching their peak.

With weeks to wait, and worried about upcoming misery, I searched the Internet on my own to see if there were any folk remedies my doctors didn't mention. Most conventional medical websites contained the same information I got when first diagnosed: the headaches are rare, they are painful and not much can be done to prevent them, except diet modification. But there was a site that was different from the others – it was called Clusterbusters.org. Basically a series of discussion boards, the site attracted hundreds of cluster headache sufferers, many who posted information about what intensified the condition, and what alleviated it.

There was one approach that seemed to consistently help people: a very small dose of psychedelic mushrooms (the kind that contain serotonin) right at the beginning of the cycle. Many sufferers claimed it broke a single cycle altogether, but many said a dose needed to be repeated when the next cycle started. Others said the mushrooms may not break the cycle, but they could relieve the pain like nothing else. Some people who were new to the boards sometimes responded that they were afraid to try psychedelic drugs. Fear wasn't a problem for me. Those kinds of drugs had already earned my respect years earlier.

The Clusterbusters did not discover medical mushrooms – researchers believe the fungus has been used in mostly non-Western cultures for thousands of years to treat a variety of maladies. And the natural health movement in the West eventually took notice. A 1980 book written by natural health guru Andrew Weil, titled *The Marriage of the Sun and the Moon*, discusses the power of mushrooms at length.

When I found the Clusterbusters site, I was married with two elementary-school age children. I hadn't sought out psychedelics for years, though I had more than my share of experience when I was younger. I had last dropped acid about nine years earlier, at a friend's bachelor party. I was introduced to the unpredictable mix of sensual pleasure and spiritual questioning that are inherent to the psychedelic experience while I and my friends were students at Northwestern University in the mid-1980s.

I had been a cannabis user for several months as a freshman, when it came time for "Armadillo Day" at the end of Spring Quarter. A campus festival of questionable origin rooted in a celebration of psychedelia, Armadillo Day was the type of event where even some professors were rumored to indulge. My first real mushroom trip was magical – it was a beautiful day with great bands and odd theatrics all geared toward mind expansion. A "chill room" with day-glo posters and toys like kaleidoscopes had been set up in the student union, and I finally understood the real value of black light. I spent the afternoon with the woman who would eventually become my wife. It was a wonderful day.

The following year, LSD (which also contains serotonin) was available around the time of Armadillo Day. A friend (who I will call "*Jack*") and I got some. We decided to take a test ride before the actual event. Knowing that it was sometimes good to have a goal in mind during a psychedelic trip, we set out on an ill-advised journey to see an X-rated movie playing in 3-D at a midnight showing at the Music Box Theater in Chicago.

It could have been a disaster. A moderate mushroom dose offered giggles over the absurdity of the commonplace with altered time and space perceptions. A full hit of LSD, as I would learn, came much closer to embodying the title of Aldous Huxley's treatise on psychedelic experience and its relationship to visionary art: *Heaven and Hell*. In the wrong time and space, a user is inviting not just strange hallucinations but the kind of raw

14

existential terror only possible when the familiar becomes alien and you feel as if you are looking at yourself from a space outside of yourself.

Huxley notes in his slender volume that a visionary experience can bring on "the horror of infinity..." While some visionaries see the world as a more beautiful place, others have the opposite experience.

"For them, as for the positive visionary, the universe is transfigured – but for the worse," Huxley writes. "Everything in it, from the stars in the sky to the dust under their feet, is unspeakably sinister or disgusting; every event is charged with hateful significance; every object manifests the presence of an Indwelling Horror, infinite, all-powerful, eternal."

At the Music Box, it wasn't all Hell, but it wasn't all Heaven. (In fact, in most of my later psychedelic experiences, it was a great deal of Heaven tinged with on occasional glimpse of Hell, but Hell sometimes gets highlighted in memory, perhaps because exceptional ugliness is easier to describe than exceptional beauty.)

I think some fellow movie-viewers may have been annoyed at our outbursts of nervous cackling over the horrible puns in the script, but the theater itself was another revelation about reality and how we perceive it. I'd been to the Music Box a few times. It was built in 1929 and retained much of its art deco charm. In the past, I found the theater to be a visually appealing place, but it never looked quite like this. There seemed to be an unusual amount of shooting stars among the night sky painted on the theater's ceiling, and the ornate facade around the screen and on the walls seemed to periodically flow into fluid motion for a moment, before regaining its familiar shape. It didn't happen when my eye was trained right on an object, but my peripheral vision was pulsing with color and light.

About 30 minutes into the movie, staying seated became

15

unbearable. I went out to the lobby where Jack was sitting on a bench and staring at the floor. He looked up, then back down at the carpet and asked if I saw it. I just nodded as I was transfixed by the sight of what seemed like a charge of visible glowing energy flowing slowly and steadily through a rounded rectangular pattern carpet. When I consciously widened my field of vision, it seemed like every single round rectangle in the carpet was swirling in unison with the visible energy that only Jack and I could see.

Such a sight might be more unnerving than entertaining to many people, especially when they realize they can't just turn it off. But that was part of the appeal to me – psychedelics, used in the right circumstances, allow the user to see something like magic, not just the magic of technology that we have now taken for granted, but sublime ancient magic that reveals beauty and depth in objects and situations that otherwise seem mundane.

And, music. Music was my special pleasure on mushrooms or acid. Listen to the right music on psychedelics – "Golden Hours" from the album *Another Green World* by Brian Eno is a favorite – and you will hear things you never expected to hear, and just sometimes, feel visceral reactions to the sounds you never may have expected.

I initially treated psychedelics as party drugs, something certain to provoke more than a few laughs. However, even when you flirt with them, they demand respect. I know people whose single psychedelic experience comprise several of the most frightening moments of their life. Disrespect can lead to psychic territory that seems uninhabitable. But, then, when you get some of the Heaven along with the Hell, even after spending time in those horribly vacant spaces, you may just find yourself more serious about looking for real meaning in the real world.

I graduated with more psychedelic experiences, but never too many to distract me from academics. I went to England to work on a student visa after college and, after a few months, fell in with another crowd that enjoyed the psychedelic experience. But, after I came home, got married and took a job as a news editor at a suburban newspaper, most of the tripping stopped, except for the odd bachelor party.

Most psychedelic drugs involve a serious time commitment – an LSD experience itself may last for 10 hours or longer. Then, for 24 hours or so, your body and mind will likely be under-performing. With adult responsibilities (particularly if you are a parent), it becomes difficult to find the time, even on weekends. So I sort of drifted away from serious trips.

I thought those days might be over altogether, until I read about the people on Clusterbusters who used psychedelics to treat cluster headaches.

When I finally saw the neurologist, he verified that I had cluster headaches. He said the standard treatment was pure oxygen, to be inhaled for several minutes right at the start of a headache. He wrote a prescription and said a tank of oxygen could be delivered to my door. Happy as I was to hear about a standard treatment, I couldn't help but ask about the mushrooms.

The neurologist said he hadn't heard of their use with cluster headaches, but given what he knew about the pain and intractability of the condition, he said he wouldn't be surprised if his patients tried almost anything that might bring relief.

4. For Your Pleasure

The oxygen helped, but it didn't stop the headaches altogether. Like most Americans in their mid-thirties, I had no idea who to call to score medicinal psychedelics. I did some research and realized home growing was possible. Then, as now, online stores offered spores of psychedelic mushrooms legally – though their use is supposed to be limited to "microscope research" according to one site.

Grow kits for any type of mushroom are also widely available. But, putting the spores into the kits and attempting to cultivate them could lead to legal trouble. Many people do grow their own, but such enterprises require sterile conditions, not the kind of down and dirty basement operation I figured I would need to hide from my family.

Once again, after the pain quieted, I almost forgot about the headaches. But, in 2006, when the next cycle started, I remembered. And I thought I knew someone who could help.

I had been writing about the consequences of the drug war and had made connections with activists, particularly in the medical cannabis community. I became friends with one, let's call him "*Roger*," who baked cannabis into cookies that were distributed to patients with Multiple Sclerosis, cancer, AIDS and other serious illnesses. My mother suffered from MS, so I bought cookies from Roger for her, and eventually for my father, when Dad was diagnosed with Parkinson's Disease and found himself unable to sleep at night.

Roger is a unique person, who shows great respect for both repeatable scientific data as well as unrepeatable spiritual experience, without finding a conflict between the two. Back then, as now, Roger reached out to friends with maladies and tried to soothe symptoms based on what he learned from accepted research. But he also tried to examine underlying stresses and problems in life which he believed can lead to disease. When I

19

told him about the headaches, and how mushrooms might help, he didn't hesitate to offer help, though he said he didn't have access to any fungus at that moment, but he would be on the lookout.

Weeks later – about halfway through the cycle – he called me. We met and he gave me a small plastic bag of stems and caps. The most experienced sufferers on Clusterbusters suggested brewing a weak tea from a small dose of mushrooms. I followed the basic instructions, which included taking the dose at the first sign of a headache.

At 3 a.m., the pain woke me. I brewed and consumed the tea according to instructions, pulled out my headphones and my old vinyl copy of *A Wizard, A True Star* by Todd Rundgren, and waited to see what happened. For one half hour, it seemed like nothing, except Todd just sounded better by the minute.

As the pain persisted I felt forlorn. As I lamented my inability to control the pain, I suddenly felt something like a channel open between the thought center in my head and the small space above my eye where the pain was concentrated. The channel seemed to offer some control over the pain, something like the volume control on the stereo I was using. I could decrease the pain by mentally dialing down the channel, though I couldn't make the pain go away altogether. And the channel also seemed able to increase the pain if I let the channel open freely, but I could quickly tone the pain back down. Uncharacteristically, well before the pain completely subsided, tears flowed from both eyes.

Happy as I was over that breakthrough, the disappointment was great when the headache returned 48 hours later, as usual, around 3 a.m. I brewed up some more tea and had a similar experience, but this time with *For Your Pleasure* by Roxy Music. I played the epic (nearly 7-minute) title track repeatedly, fascinated as it unraveled from a vocal accompanied by piano into an echo-laden otherworldly spasm of sound that slowly diffuses into the universe. I felt good and eventually went back to bed to sleep well.

Three nights later, when the pain woke me up, I felt too tired to get up, so I just took a small piece of the mushroom and placed it under my tongue. I think I perceived that nothing was happening for several moments, but the next thing I knew, it was 7 a.m., and unlike most other headache nights, I felt rested. The thought of getting up didn't seem nearly as bad as it usually did after a headache.

I knew the cycle was waning anyway, but I'd never had an experience like that before. Just going back to sleep may not sound like an exceptional thing, but for years, I simply could not sleep through the headaches, and this time I seemed to. It was also counter-intuitive that the mushroom, even a tiny bit, would put me to sleep. I always found the inability to sleep at the end of a psychedelic experience a downside, but the tiny dose of mushroom actually did put me back to sleep.

I repeated the process over the next couple weeks, until the headaches were just shadows. I had three decent size mushrooms left. I wasn't sure how long they would keep without losing their potency, but I wanted to keep a little bit for next time, so I saved one.

The other two were used when Jack and I went to see Pink Floyd guitarist David Gilmore at the Rosemont Theatre. It was a much bigger dose than I was used to, but not huge, and I tripped out a bit on the beauty of whole mushrooms themselves, as opposed to fragments. If you were at the show, you may have noticed me. I was the idiot in back yelling for more lasers.

5. Feeling Yourself Disintegrate

As always, when the cycle started 3 years later, I was a bit startled and surprised, but I felt ready. I still had one mushroom left, and when I called Roger, he said he could get more. I never made the tea again. I used the Small Piece Under Tongue method. I thought I discovered it, but on Clusterbusters it is well-known and sometimes referred to by acronym (SPUT).

A SPUT, along with the oxygen prescribed by the doctor, usually had me back to sleep in 20 minutes or so with early headaches, with the pain diminishing well before its typical peak. But, the cycle followed its usual pattern, with frequency and intensity increasing dramatically after a month. The smaller pieces of mushrooms weren't as effective, so I started using bigger pieces.

I met with Roger to get more mushrooms. We chatted over lunch. He had learned more about cluster headaches, and the medicinal possibilities of psychedelics. He said he had seen a sufferer of persistent cluster headaches break their cycle with one full dose of LSD and a smaller follow up dose. He had also been watching for more information about the condition, and discovered that a Harvard researcher had surveyed cluster headache sufferers and found that more found relief through psychedelics than any conventional treatment, including oxygen. (The researcher, John Halpern, has since started a corporation called Entheogen to devise a cure for cluster headaches based on some components of psychedelic drugs.)

I told Roger how the mushrooms were working to relieve pain, but that the cycle was progressing as usual. He said he would get the mushrooms, but he also offered to get some acid and host me at his place for the 12 hours or so I would need for the trip.

Much as I was ready to try anything for more relief, the idea wasn't an automatic slam dunk with me. I remembered that a

23

trip to Heaven doesn't preclude a detour to Hell. My experience with heavier psychedelics told me that they tended to make everything more intense. What if one of the headaches started on the acid, but then became overly intense? As we talked in a northside diner, a cover version of one of my favorite Flaming Lips song – "Feeling Yourself Disintegrate" performed by a band I still don't know – started playing on the sound system. It seemed to be a good omen, and I was reminded of the one time a headache cycle ended well before its time.

I was in England just after college, and about one month into the visit, I think the headaches started. Of course, that was before the headaches had been diagnosed, but I remember waking up and thinking I needed sinus medicine, which was my automatic response to the headaches at that time. I had to go to the local chemist and find sinus pills. I found them and used them for about a week, but then I didn't need to use them anymore. I'm pretty sure the headaches disappeared after one of my new friends in England had obtained some acid and shared a full dose with me during a night of clubbing.

That memory sealed the deal – if it worked before, maybe it would work again. I was ready to take my first acid trip in roughly a decade.

6. It's All Too Much

It's impossible to convey exactly what happens in an LSD experience, especially one that was sort of focused like this one was, other than to say it was good. I didn't have a headache during the trip. I stayed more or less by myself listening to music, thinking and perceiving. Reflecting afterward, I realized I was coming to terms with having more real responsibilities in my life. My kids were growing older, but so were my parents, and somehow the trip made me realize it was up to me to be responsive to their needs even when we had a hard time communicating about those needs.

In a strange but significant moment the next day, I walked by my then 13-year-old daughter's room. My favorite Beatles song – "It's All Too Much" (which I believe captures the psychedelic experience more profoundly than any of their other songs, including "I am the Walrus") was playing on my daughter's radio. She asked if everything was OK – she said my wife had told her that I needed to take a day to work on headaches. In my semi-coherent post-trip haze, it was all too much just for a moment, but then my mind came together and we talked about it for a while (without specifically mentioning LSD), and it was OK. Shortly after that, I went over to my parents' place and, for the first time in my life, told them about a psychedelic experience. They understood.

The headaches stayed away for about 24 hours, but about 36 hours after the acid trip, I had the worst headache of the cycle. It was like the pain had no power during acid time, but when that protection was gone, the pain struck back with a vengeance. The intensity of the headaches started diminishing right after that, but I still used a little piece of mushroom to get through the more intense ones in the final weeks. The LSD trip didn't really work the way I envisioned, but like most psychedelic experiences, it probably happened just the way it should have.

7. I've Been Born Again

Once again, after the last headache of the last cycle, I started to forget. Indeed, for 3 years after the last headache, nothing happened. But part way through that fourth year, I was awakened by a twinge at about 3 a.m. on a mild November morning. That's when I crept down to the garage, got the stepladder, and pulled out the mushrooms that were left from the last time. I placed a small piece under my tongue, and indeed, I was back to sleep in minutes.

A few nights later, I took a bigger dose, maybe four times what I usually take. It wasn't meant to be a serious trip, but it was supposed to blast the cycle away. Unfortunately, it did not. Another headache came back in a few days. I called Roger.

He said he and his colleagues had been using LSD in a new way. They would take roughly one-tenth of a traditional dose of the drug. The experience was somewhat shorter and definitely less intense, he said. Next time I saw him, he gave me a sheet of paper that contained several of the "tenners."

A few days later, when I felt a headache come on, I took one of the tenners. As predicted, it was shorter (about 7 hours) and much less intense, but still thought provoking. I hung around the house with my family, and acted more or less normally, with just a few moments when I became unusually interested in common objects. At the end, I felt a sense of peace I never felt at the end of a full-blown trip. The headache didn't come back for a few days, but then it seemed less intense. Within about 6 weeks, instead of the traditional minimum of 3 months, the headaches were gone altogether.

I don't know if or when the pain will come back, but I remain armed with knowledge. I may have turned on and tuned in, a la Timothy Leary, but in my case, the acid may have prevented me from dropping out.

The whole experience has failed to change me from the middle-aged suburbanite I evolved into after college. My wife and I have jobs to pay the mortgage, the kids go to school – we even go to church with some regularity. And when I am in the sanctuary, I frequently but quietly thank God for the underground drug culture that not only brought a special kind of joy to my life, but just might have saved it.

Appendix
Suggested Listening

Chapter 1 – Any performance of John Cage's 4' 33"
Chapter 2 – Side 4 of "Metal Machine Music" by Lou Reed
Chapter 3 – "Golden Hours" by Brian Eno
Chapter 4 – "For Your Pleasure" by Roxy Music
Chapter 5 – "Feeling Yourself Disintegrate" by Flaming Lips
Chapter 6 – "It's All Too Much" by The Beatles
Chapter 7 – "I've Been Born Again" by Jessy Dixon and the
                   Chicago Community Choir

www.ingramcontent.com/pod-product-compliance
Lightning Source LLC
Chambersburg PA
CBHW060352290526
45791CB00004B/1640